MY JOURNEY TO 2020

Pia Lord
THE PIA LORD COMPANY

My Journey to 2020

From Multiple Vision to

"Perfect" Vision

by
Pia Lord

Dedication

To my son Rex,
I so wish to see the world with you growing up in it.

Acknowledgements

I would like to thank my parents, Martha and Kurt Fiedler for their generous donations to my surgery, and encouragement to write, without which this book and my new 20/20 eyesight would not have happened in a timely manner. Thank you also to friends in the Everglades who persuaded me to just have the surgery done, when I couldn't see what they were seeing on a guided tour! Thank you to the medical professionals at the Eye Institute for Medicine and Surgery in Melbourne, Florida whose guidance and specialties made this all possible. Finally, thank you to my family for their support throughout the process.

Table of Contents

Introduction

Chapter 1............... Types of Vision Issues

Chapter 2............... Night Swimming and Noticing Changes

Chapter 3............... Steadily Decreasing and Changing Vision-Pictures

Chapter 4................. Doctors' Visits

Chapter 5................. Early Cataracts-Understanding the Disease

Chapter 6................. The Hope of Home Remedies

Chapter 7................... From Ambivalence to Firm Resolve

Chapter 8................. The Procedure and Recovery Protocol

Chapter 9................. The 30-Day Post Surgery Journal

Chapter 10............... The Reward of Restored Eyesight and Return to Productive Life

'Never say 'no' to adventures. Always say 'yes,' otherwise you'll lead a very dull life. '

—<u>Ian Fleming</u>

Introduction

When I was a young girl, I marveled at the world through clear eyes and good corrected vision. I was happy to travel the world and see interesting sights such as the Eiffel Tower, the Temple of Nike, the Acropolis, Munich Biergartens, Verona's House of Capulets, La Scala, Rome, NYC, Mykonos, Berling, Lac d'Annecy, the Metropolitan Opera House and stroll on the Kurferstendam in Berlin. Fast forward 20-30 years and gradually my vision deteriorated to near blindness, multiple vision and cataract development. Fortunately, I had clear close vision and night vision. I was able to see through my double and triple images of the moon and car headlights because intellectually I knew what it was supposed to be. Hence, I was coping via knowledge of 30 years of correctly seeing while driving. I always relied upon the knowledge that incorrect vision could be corrected via glasses and contacts. But one day I went to the optometrist and she said my left eye could not be correct to 20/20 any longer. This is the story of my vision, vision loss, and return to sight through the technology in modern ophthalmology. It has been a scary last two years of my life realizing that my vision was deteriorating into blindness and upsetting by not seeing my son in his winter concert band performance, although I was in the audience. I am writing this book out of gratitude for my new vision. If you too suffer vision loss, I hope to help you and encourage you to seek professional help sooner than later and to have courage. My parents also had cataract removal and Intraocular Lens (IOL) implantation surgeries. Fortunately, due to the success of both of their eye operations, I eventually mustered the courage to go ahead with the process. I was driving without realizing how much detail in my vision I had lost. Only upon having a new lens implantation done can I compare the amount of detail I lost and the degree to which I was coping in my everyday activities. Throughout this decline, I was truly hoping for a miracle since surgery was the last thing, I thought I could undergo. I tried many things from supplements for eyes to smoothies and prayer. The true miracle it turns out has been the advances in ophthalmic technology and the skills of the surgeon in replacing my lenses. Nevertheless, I still pray to have faith and courage to go through with the procedures and the patience to listen to the doctor's orders when they tell a swimmer and kayaker that she can't be on or in the water for a whole month!

I truly hope that if your vision is deteriorating or if you know of someone that has cataracts, this book can help them know what's ahead in the process. In this book I share with you the two years of declining vision. Pass on the knowledge that cataract surgery is not as scary as I once thought. Finding an excellent eye institute, having great guidance with doctors, and following the procedures suggested lead to restored eyesight. In the chapters of this book, I include a daily journal on the progression of my vision from the day of surgery to one month later including the behaviors that I practiced assuring a proper surgical outcome. I hope to have erred on the side of overprotection, all the while trying to not be bored "playing it safe" following doctors' orders.

I assume if you are still reading this you or someone you know, do have eye issues that need to be resolved. So, I wish you best guidance, patience and dutifulness in attending to your vision restoration. Best of luck to you. If I can help in any way, please email me at pialord@gmail.com or connect with me on Facebook at PiaLord. Here's to many more years of travel and seeing our world!

Chapter 1

Types of Vision Issues

I started having numerous vision issues besides the regular declining of overall general eyesight. The different types of vision issue I started having included multiple vision with lights at night, dimming vision, blurred vision in left eye, shadowing of lettering, then blurring of vision in right eye, binoculars with clear vision and split images of 5 or more in right eye and 3 in left eye. This caused me an enormous amount of stress as these types of issues affected first my left eye and later my right eye. I felt like it was okay if both eyes were not affected. But once both eyes were showing signs of deterioration, I started to get very worried. Multiple vision is the phenomenon where there is more than one of the same image present. Multiple vision with lights at night is best described by looking at a stop light and seeing two red lights next to each other, even overlapping like a Venn diagram circles, when there is, only one. In my case, the multiple vision was only present at night with lights, at first. Later, the splitting lights or multiple lights occurred during the daytime too. Farther into this vision loss, ordinary objects started having shadows and doubling too. It took about a year for trees, cars, houses, poles, people to look like there were two of those also.

Dimming vision can be described by needing more and more light to see the same things I used to see. At one point, I thought our house was getting so dark. We had not added or subtracted any lamps in any rooms, but the ambient light never seemed to be enough to see properly. Another example is when I was in my car, the inside car lights appeared to be dim. I had to increase the back light on my phone gradually to 100 percent. When we moved to Florida and bought a new house with white tile floors, I became very frustrated because they always were looking more and more yellow. The yellowing of the white is a sign of cataract. Another example from driving is that if I was driving on a single lane road, I would need to put on my high beams just to see the road in front of me at night. Sometimes this really bothered oncoming cars and even cars I happen to be following. So, I would switch on and off my high beams, trying to be courteous, all the while just trying to see the road ahead.

    Blurred vision in my left eye started to occur after I had a piece of wood jump into my eye once when I was gardening. The pain was excruciating, and I had an emergency visit to the ophthalmologist in NJ. He removed the tiny piece of wood and said there was a bit of abrasion on the cornea. Apart from that everything was fine. At least the pain was gone. My left eye always needed a stronger prescription than the right eye. So naturally I assumed it was just a matter of course that my vision became fuzzier in the left eye first. Images were no longer sharp and clear. Letters on a black board were blurred together and hazy. At back to school night, it took me forever to read the teachers email address on the whiteboard, so I missed writing it down before the next PowerPoint slide came up. So, I was slow in communicating with my son's teachers.

    Shadowing of lettering occurred more and more. I will describe this in a few different ways. The shadow of a letter is when the bold original letter is followed by a lighter version of the same letter. Hence you get a word that will be written with doubled letters. In addition, this same phenomenon can occur not just to the right, but also above the original word, or to the left or below. One time I was looking at a sign and a double image of the letters of the sign appeared. The image was crystal clear. I thought my vision had improved immediately. Then I noticed that it was a doubled vision. Hence two lines of text above and below with the upper one being clear and the lower blurred. This issue made reading road signs difficult unless I already knew what the sign said. Familiarity with my environment helped me to be able to function although I was really seeing such distorted images. I knew that I had to seek further medical attention though when although familiar with roads, the white side lines were doubling and cars ahead of me were also doubling. Oncoming cars at night looked like a maze of headlights. Sometimes there were three lights for every single light of a headlight. So, if I had an oncoming car there would be six yellowish headlights staring at me. I knew of course to stay in my lane, but to avoid such large amount of light approaching me I would slightly avert my gaze into the dark of the night. The mass of lights made driving more and more stressful to the point that I started telling my husband and friends and family that I no longer drive at night. This started to put a damper on my life!

For about a year from about January 2017 to January 2018 the split vision was only in my left eye. Sometimes it was fun to see three or five red lights at a stop light and marvel about how it always looked like Christmas. I think it was in the winter of February 2018. But then one night I opened my right eye and closed my left eye, while at a stop light. It was then that I noticed that the multiple vision was also occurring in my right eye. The split lights would occur with white light first, then red, green, and yellow lights. The streetlights had halos and looked like snowflakes. My eyes were reacting differently to light at this point. The failing in my left eye had gone to multiples of three to five sometimes more, depending upon how late at night it was or how tired I was. The right eye was only splitting the images and lights into two more or less identical shapes. When I put my glasses on, the splitting would diminish to somewhat normal vision. After our move to Florida, perhaps with the increased sun in the wintertime, the vision challenges started accelerating. In December of 2018, I was at my son's winter concert sitting in the audience and I started to cry. I could see a blur of the band, I could hardly see his trombone section with the three trombones, and I could not make him out clearly. This was probably the most upsetting moment of my entire vision loss period of my life. Here my son was just getting to be a teenager. I did not want to start going blind currently in his life.

On a recent trip during Christmas of 2018, my husband was driving, and it had gotten to be nighttime. We were on 95 North heading towards Raleigh Durham to visit relatives. I had the binoculars in the glove compartment and got them out to test my vision. Since I was not convinced from the latest eye appointment that I should need surgery, I was constantly testing my own vision to see if it was getting better or worse. Speeding along at 70 mph, I could barely read signs as we approached and passed them by without my glasses or even with my glasses. So, I place the binoculars in front of my eyes to see what might happen. In other eye appointments, doctors had told me my retina was clear, my cornea was fine, and I had no other issues but cataracts. But I was only 50 years old and I never saw any whitening in my pupil sometimes present in cataracted eyes. Well, through the binoculars I could see perfectly clearly, at night. There were no multiple images! So, this led me thinking all over again that maybe I did not have cataracts but something else. Why could I see clearly with binoculars and not without? Perhaps if doctors just gave me binocular glasses then I'd be fine. Or perhaps the eyeglasses prescription was misdiagnosed.

Split images of 3 or more in right eye and 5 in left eye started to occur after January 2019. I had studied astrophysics and gotten my M.S. in Space Studies. I had become very interested in telescopes and viewing the night sky. However, I realized that I would have to give up nighttime viewing as the moon now was a conglomeration of 5 interlocking and overlapping circles of various shades of white and silver. I would never be able to distinguish any planets or stars properly again. I just gave up.

When my husband wanted to go out and see the rocket launches from Cape Canaveral, even from our front sidewalk, I would go but became increasingly discouraged as I could not clearly see the rocket. Friends wanted to play music and go kayaking, I declined because I constantly had to put the music so close to my face, they began to take notice. Even with glasses everything was a blurry mess. I stopped playing piano at home because even reading the music became so difficult. I had to slide the music rack very far forward and still could not see the notes. Playing hymns, which I do well became somewhat of a farce! Wrong notes in chords do not sound great in very familiar hymns. Kayaking still was doable because it is largely a large muscle group exercise. The area in which I live is pretty much foolproof for not getting lost. The Indian River Lagoon has two sides and a straight body of water. Not many places to get lost if you just follow the coastline! I was able to still paddle alone 15 miles at my longest 4-hour training. That was a Godsend!

Chapter 2

Night Swimming and Noticing Changes

Since 1997, I had participated on and off in open water swimming. My first 1-mile swim was at Todd's Point in Greenwich, Connecticut. I did it for fun because I thought it would be a challenge to swim in the Long Island Sound. I began to increase my training in a pool until I could swim 10k doing pool laps. Then I felt confident to do more open water swims such as swimming in Mallorca, coastal swims off of Tenerife, swimming island to island in the British Virgin Islands (5K) as well as swimming Lido Key (15K), swimming across the Chesapeake Bay (10K) and lake swimming in Colorado and Vermont (5-10K). The heavy chlorine in the pools where I trained had a negative drying effect on my skin, my lungs and I think my eyes. Nevertheless, I was enchanted with the idea of Returning to the Sea as a human being, claiming or reclaiming the vast territory of the oceans as a swimmer, doing no harm to the life therein. I wrote a series of books Return to the Sea and Return to the Sea II. But the one problem among many in doing so is that seeing under the sea is very fuzzy. Sighting while swimming, looking where you are going amidst the waves, the choppy waters, the windy conditions is a definite skill required in the open water. Staying on course and holding your own, navigating while swimming (as fish might) requires quite good eyesight. Swimming with prescription goggles of diopter -6 helped me tremendously. With new goggles, I was able to easily swim the coastal areas of Mallorca and sight well in swimming from Norman Island (BVI)- to Flanigan Island (USVI). But after a while the goggles fog up, get scratched and become useless. Then it's time for a new pair. The combination of developing cloudy cataracted lenses with scratched googles became perplexing. I was not able to sight properly anymore. I participated in an Ocean City Games swim of 9 miles straight along the coast. I ended up swimming practically in circles, towards the beach, and against the current. I didn't even make it to the first check point in time at 3 miles before I was pulled out of the race. Whether it was the conditions or my eyes, or the combination, that race was a DNF for sure. What boggled my mind was that this race was a straight coastal swim, following the curve of the land the entire way and I could not do it. I simply was not swimming or sighting in a straight line. I really was not sighting at all. I plain could not see the next condo building unless it was right next to me. My vision had become so blurred that it really hampered my sighting ability in open water. Without a decent kayaker to guide my swim I had no hope of swimming for the mark miles in the distance. So, into my life walks Don McCumber, captain of Diana Nyad's kayaker team in her swim from Cuba to Key West. He has an innate or highly developed sense of direction, understanding of the wave patterns, currents, and how to properly navigate in all conditions. With his guidance, I was able to swim to Alligator Lighthouse and back, from buoy to buoy, even though I could not see the next buoy, a quarter of a mile in the distance. While I was dodging jellyfish, he was leading the course. I stayed next to his kayak and just swam. When I deviated, he would call me over and I'd swim back to the kayak. Even though the swim buoy were enormous, I still could not see them from in the water with my eyes. He gently guided me around the course and thus I was able to complete this swim.

The excellent sighting ability I once had deteriorated rapidly once the cataract set in and began to grow, clouding my vision.

Chapter 3

Steadily Decreasing and Changing Vision

Pictures of the Moon

From 2009 to 2012 I was studying for my Master of Science degree in Space Science Studies. I bought a telescope, began star gazing, went to a few star parties, and attended a Star conference in Astronomy in St. Louis, Missouri. I was excited about lunar geology, solar physics and the blossoming field of satellite communications. I would set up the telescope on my lawn and from there I could clearly see the moon, lunar craters, and lunar mare. In my trips back and forth to the pool as a member of Lifetime Fitness from 2013 to 2018, I would see the different phases of the moon very clearly driving on Route 78 in New Jersey. Sometimes I would see the harvest moon in its enormity. Other times I saw the moon in waxing or waning gibbous phase. And other times I saw just the small sliver of a silvery crescent or the second quarter moon. I was excited about possibly working in the field of lunar exploration or SATCOM. One night after swim training, I was driving and saw a double moon. I thought it was odd. So, I closed my right eye and sure enough there were two crescents overlapping each other. One was the bright moon and the secondary was the multiple in shadowy form that my cataract had created. I thought it was cool at first. I closed my left eye and briefly looked at the moon with my right eye. There was just one moon. I felt safe and okay. I knew that I could function fine with my dominant eye, my right eye being clear. I swam regularly and over the course of a year and a half, I noticed changes occurring in my left eye. These changes included more multiple images going from 2-5-7 images of an object, especially the moon. I was basically tracking my decline in vision as I was enamored and disturbed by the things my eyes were doing. I continued driving, albeit slower since I wanted to have a better safety net in case my eyes presented me with a picture my mind could not unscramble fast enough. Month by month, I would see differences in the images my left eye was taking in. In addition to the increasing number of overlapping images, I was also experiencing progressive blurriness. There was also a web like veil over any images I was getting from my left eye.

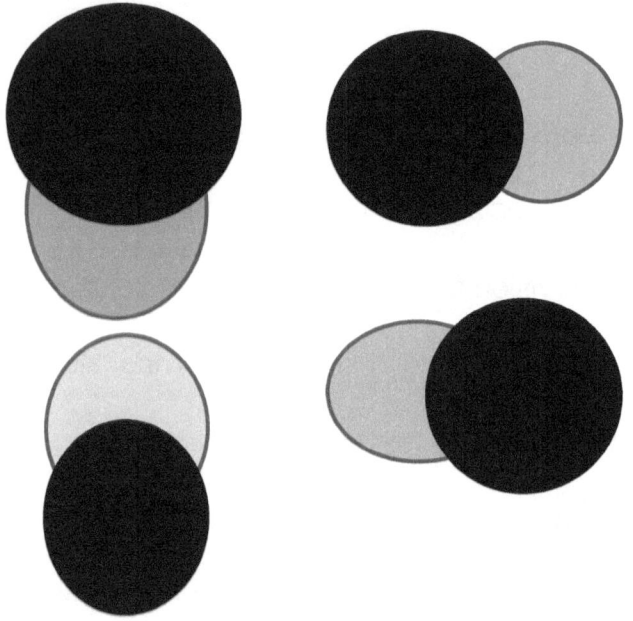

The images I was seeing could be doubled above, below, to the left and to the right. As the vision grew worse, the multiples went around the original image in a circular way. The first drawing below, on the left, was my vision with my glasses on. When I removed my glasses, I would see so many more multiples.

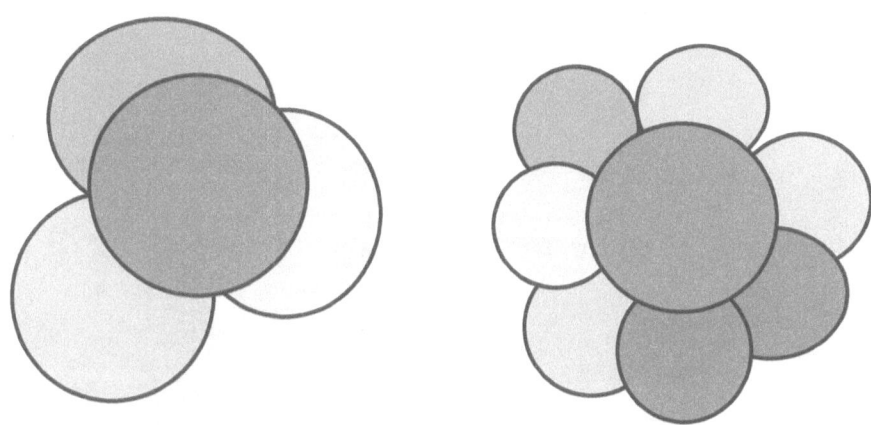

Darkest grey circle represents original image of moon, stop light, headlight, streetlight or even the sun.

The next interesting image set that I got was a blurred line of text with an extremely clear line of text above. It looks somewhat like this. The text is the same, the positioning of the double is either directly above the original text or it was shifted to the right above the original text line.

I see this line extremely clearly

I see this line completely blurred

Seeing the top text so clearly gave me hope that my eyes were getting better. But I was not able to eliminate the blurry bottom text. This situation only happened a couple of times while I was driving on Rt. 520, a main road near my house looking at the store signs. The actual business sign did not say the above text. But this represents the text as I saw it.

The next very noticeable worsening of my vision came while driving on the road to my house. I had oncoming cars with headlights on. I saw triple images for every headlight. When cars were in the distance and I could see 5 car headlights at once, then each headlight was also tripled. So, I was seeing 30 lights when there were only 5 sets of lights or 10 lights. Not only were there so many more lights but each light had halos around them. I was seeing a mass of overlapping lights. I then saw this type of image for a period of approximately 5-6 months. I was able to manage the images up to a point and still drive. It was mainly my left eye that created the triple, but my right eye soon followed and was creating triple images sometimes and doubles others. But when the eyes work together, I was seeing the triple. This would occur at any lights, stop lights, Christmas lights at houses, headlights, house lights, streetlights. Thank goodness I have a great brain as I was able to sort out the actual light from the triples. However, as this situation developed it became overwhelming and stressful. I knew that I could not continue to function in driving a car if this became any worse. On another local trip, shortly thereafter, I realized that at one moment, my brain became confused with these images. I think my left eye dominated at that time and in this switch from left eye dominate to right eye dominate, I had a momentary visual perception overload in which my driving knowledge was superseded by a new sensory overload. I was able to blink, shake my head and remain in control. But at this time, I knew that I had to find a true solution to my vision problems.

Chapter 4

Doctors' Visits

In New Jersey, I went to the Essex Eye Institute for a checkup and usually obtained my glasses from Costco, or Pearl Vision. One time I went to the Essex Eye Institute, was seen by an optometrist who said that my left eye could no longer be correct to 20/20. I then went to Retina Specialists in Essex County and found there was no issue with the retina. I also went to a Corneal Specialist, Dr. Childs in Montclair and was told my corneas were fine too.

In Maryland, where my parents had cataract surgery and IOL implantation done, I was seen by an associate in Dr Maria Scott's office in Annapolis, MD. It was recommended at the age of 48, for me to have cataract removal and lens implantation as well as glaucoma surgery. My parents would not let me have the surgery through this office because they thought I was too young. They had lens implantation at the ages of 82 and 85.

In Florida, I went to the Walmart Vision Center and had my eyes checked. My eye glass prescription was increased from -5.5 to -6.5 in the left eye and -5.5 to -6.0 in the right eye. Even at the optometrist's office my vision was still blurred. When I received the eyeglasses a few weeks later, they did not help much. I was referred to the Florida Eye Institute. I made one appointment and cancelled; I was so scared. I next asked friends and family for another referral for a good ophthalmologist. My brother and sister in law recommended that I try prism glasses first. So, I sought out a multiple vision specialist to get a pair of prism glasses. This led me to Dr. Mandese, an optometrist at the Eye Institute for Medicine and Surgery in Melbourne, Florida. I had one appointment with him. He recommended cataract surgery immediately. He explained to me that his analysis determined that prism glasses would not help me because there was nothing wrong with the musculature surrounding my eyes and that my eyes were functioning normally. He did say that the reason for my multiple vision was due to the cataracts in both eyes.

Chapter 5

Early Cataracts-Understanding the Disease

Understanding my visual situation took visits to the doctor and a lot of listening and learning on my part. At the Eye Institute, my optometrist explained to me how the clear normal human lens allows light to enter the eye, focus on the retina, produce an image on the brain and process the information. He explained that when the lens gets clouded the light cannot enter, multiple images get formed due to scattering of light. I understood that the light was not focusing to produce one image, rather I had a lot of scattering of light occurring which produced the myriad of images I was seeing. Upon my request he took pictures of my lens which looked whitish and yellowish.

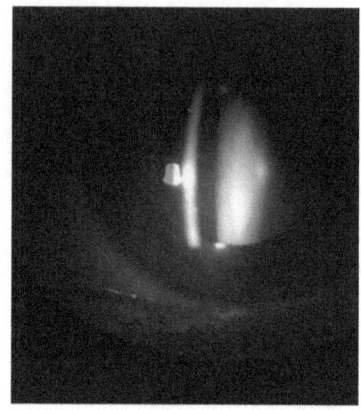

Figure 1 Left Eye Cataract

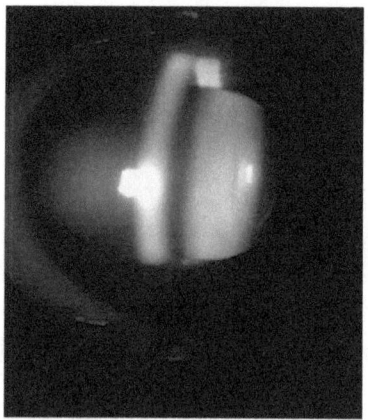

Figure 2 Right Eye Cataract

After my first visit, the next day I had an appointment with Dr. Jason Darlington, ophthalmologist-cataract removal and IOL implantation specialist. After confirming the cataracts, he explained my options, including single focal lens, multi-focal lens, one of each in either eye, doing nothing, and time frames. He mentioned that the surgeries are usually done one to two weeks apart to give the eyes time to adjust. He showed me a large size demonstration model of the Intraocular Lens by Johnson and Johnson Labs, the Symphony Multi-focal lens. The demonstration model lens was interesting in that it was a series of concentric circles which created the possibility of 20/20 vision at every distance, depending upon how the eye would work with it and adjust to it. He said that with the single focus lens, I would have clear distance vision but everything else would be blurry and I would need glasses. Implanting the multi-focal lens would give me mostly clear vision at arm's length, and clear mid and distance vision.

The following visit was for scheduling and measuring my eyes. An ophthalmic technician took measurements and then I visited with a surgical counselor for over an hour to set up the entire surgical and follow up visits. The next time I would return would be for the first surgery.

Chapter 6

The Hope of Home Remedies

I went home from my scheduling meeting with the surgical counselor and furiously looked online for other solutions. Although I had scheduled all my surgeries and post-operative follow up appointments, I still wanted to avoid eye surgery. Over the years I looked for alternative medicine treatments to failing vision. I did eye exercises, drank smoothies, and stocked up on beta carotene, collagen, gingko biloba, bilberry, cinnamon, Occuvite, vitamins A, C, E, Zinc, lutein, lutein blue, zeaxanthin, alpha lipoic acid and every other possible available over the counter supplement. The more supplements the industry came out with the more I tried them. But I rarely bought more than one container, except of beta carotene, lutein, zeaxanthin and bilberry since none of them provided the solution that I was looking for. I had some betterment in my visual acuity using beta carotene and bilberry, but in the end, my vision never cleared or returned to 20/20 using any of the supplements. I also read about drops for dog cataracts which apparently work; however, I did not venture into that area. I also began eating a lot more carrots thinking I would try the natural nutritional way. I think eating proper vegetables does help in supporting my eyes, but at 54, it did not bring back 20/20 vision, clear the cataracts or eliminate the multiple vision I was having. I did read about eye drops containing l- carnitine, marigold and other herbs. I tried certain teas also which might support vision, but these too did not prevent me from getting more blind in my left eye and experiencing decreasing vision in my right eye. I read that the l-carnitine drops were helping people's vision at least as far as the reviews on the product website. However, these people had to continue to apply drop for months to years at a time, continually purchasing the product. I considered that the surgery would be an easier and more final solution.

Chapter 7

From Ambivalence to Firm Resolve

My next appointment was a scheduling appointment for surgery at the Eye Institute. I spent three hours with Lisa, the surgical counselor. I scheduled left eye surgery, one day follow up, one week follow up appointments. I scheduled right eye surgery, one day post op, one-week post operative follow up appointments. My intention was to get going with this process on a superficial level. I would schedule the appointments, then go home and find a true home remedy that worked. Then I would cancel the surgery, having restored my vision all by myself! My idea was to schedule the surgery for one month out to give me time to do more research and look for other online sources that promised and delivered solutions to cataract vision issues. I had found a surgeon researcher in India that promise restored vision via a special surgical procedure and one in Russia who developed a solution with L-carnitine eye drops.

However, God must have had another plan for me! My "best laid plans" and this schedule did not happen. The surgical counselor and I set dates for the following two weeks. I had become curious about the phacoemulsification procedure and if it could really work for me as it had for my parents and two other women that I talked to on a boat trip in the Everglades. These ladies and I were visiting Jewel Key with Everglades Area Tours head guide and manager, Captain Don McCumber. Don pointed out raccoons on the outer island near Chokoloskee, Florida. The ladies both said they saw the raccoons and even pointed out other racoons too on a neighboring island. I tried hard to see them, but I never did. They said I should look out for movement on the ground. I was so embarrassed to admit that I could not see them. I even got angry inside of myself because I was an ACA Level 3 Coastal Kayaking Trip Leader and I could not do what I had taking training for due to my eyes. I then asked the ladies who were at least (in their 70s) twenty years older than me how they could see so well! They replied that they both had lens replacement surgery in both eyes! I was awestruck! I was convinced on the spot! I went from skeptical hesitation to anticipation of my surgery in about one second! I then knew that this was my solution and I stopped looking for other home remedies. I went back home and ordered my eye drops and planned for my first eye surgery the next week.

Chapter 8

The Procedure and Recovery Protocol

The Procedure

The ophthalmic surgery procedure that I had done is phacoemulsification with IOL implantation. Phacoemulsification is basically the breaking up or emulsification of the natural albeit cataracted lens with an ultrasonic handpiece and then aspirated from the eye. Aspirated fluids are replaced with irrigation of balanced salt solution to maintain the anterior chamber. An intraocular lens is then implanted into the eye. Phaco-emulsification is the most common cataract surgery performed.

It is used to restore vision which has become distorted due to the clouding of the eye lens.

A special multi-focal lens was selected by my doctor for each eye, according to measurements taken and a computer algorithm. These silicone lenses are implanted behind the cornea into the casing where the natural lens used to be. The surgery prep involves four rounds of local anesthesia and iodine drops, along with a needle in the left hand to inject a calming agent for nerves. After the local anesthesia has been applied, cold water is poured over the surgical area. The iodine drops determine if the area is numbed sufficiently. The multi-focal lenses by Symphony from Johnson and Johnson cost $2600 per lens. The surgeon fees for this 15-minute operation itself cost over $3000 for both eyes. My insurance did not cover the cost of the lenses nor the procedure. My rational was that to buy new eyeglasses which cost $400 every 8 months would eventually be much costlier than to pay for this process now. I am told that these lenses last a lifetime. I am 54 years old and my parents are 90. So, I estimate that these lenses will last another 40 years. I do wonder about having silicone in my eyes for 40 years. But so far, they are very comfortable and do not feel very different from my normal lenses. I can adjust to 20/20!

Recovery Protocol

One day prior to surgery 3 different eye drops are required three times per day, morning, noon and nighttime. The day of surgery one drop of each solution is required in the morning. The drops need to be administered 3 minutes apart. My ophthalmic solution drops were Moxifloxacin, Prednisolone Acetate and Ketorolac Tromethamine. The day of surgery, after the procedure, the drops need to be administered every two hours until bedtime. Truly this is a very time-consuming process. In addition, the daily schedule of 3 drops, 3 times per day continues for 28 days. It is very important to follow this regime consistently. I used the check off sheet to make sure that I did not skip any applications of the drops. My doctor father and nurse mother reinforced the importance of sticking to the application of all drops and getting an extra supply of the drops so I would not run out in the middle of the night. The drops cost $118 for three tiny bottles at CVS. The total for the drops is $236 so far. I still have one refill good until March 15, 2020!

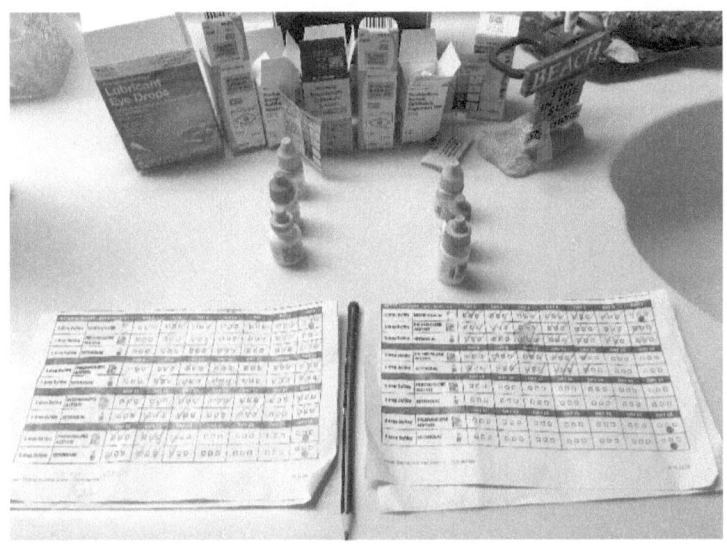
Figure 3 Eye Drop Station

I set up an eye drop station in my bathroom. This was going to be a long process of protocol and recovery. These two eyes drop check lists were for my right and lefts eyes and each for 28 days. One day pre-operative and day of surgery eye drop procedures are included. As you can see, I hope, I follow the doctor's orders dutifully, and check off each time I put in the eye drops.

Chapter 9

The 30-Day Post Surgery Journal

(February 22-March 22, March 5- April 5, 2019)

Day 1 2/22/2019 Left Eye Surgery Whitish light in front of objects. Still blurred vision. I was amazed how everything that looked yellowish with my right eye, now was pure white with my left eye new lens. I began to understand how much my vision had deteriorated from a normal healthy eye and vision. Left eye vision had no doubled objects or multiple vision.

Day 2 Clear sharp highly detailed far vision. I was very happy with this new lens for seeing details long distance. In driving I no longer had any multiple vision with my left eye. But up-close vision was not yet clear.

Day 3 I was reading my piano music again from a normal distance on the music rack of my Steinway. Sitting at my computer reading the screen was easy again, with my left eye dominating the vision. But holding my phone with regular font, not bold was illegible. I changed to bold and then with increasing the size of the font slightly I could make out the words.

Day 4 I was still basically relying on my right eye to read up close print on my phone and any letters, magazines or papers. I went to a small museum and was able to read the caption under the exhibits from a normal distance. This I had not been able to do in a long time.

Day 5 For the next five days until I went in for the surgery on my right eye, I was comparing the clear, clean vision in my left eye with the yellowing, blurry, multiple vision that I was still seeing in my right eye.

Day 6 I was contemplating the second surgery very seriously. I had already signed up for it but was reluctant to lose my very good up-close vision still working in my right eye. The doctor said that I would have close (arm's length), mid distance (computer distance) and far vision. The up-close vision I had with my right eye allowed me to hold my phone about 4 inches from my face and see very clearly. I could play mini pool, check Gmail, text, go on Facebook, go on golf app, do basically anything I wanted to do. But I was concerned that I was holding the iPhone or the Samsung too close to my face. So, I was willing to forgo this good vision that I had left and opt for good distance and mid-distance vision with possibility of having some up-close vision. I realized that I could easily switch to a tablet and just slightly increase the font to achieve easier healthier reading vision.

Day 7 2/28/2019 Now it has been one week since my lens implantation. I was grateful for the advances in modern medicine and my new sight.

Day 8 3/1/2019 I had one bit of pain at night in my left ear. I think it had to do with playing my flute. It did not affect my vision.

Day 9 Thought about how I want to do a TED TALK and finish writing this book to help other people who are struggling with their vision. I thought it could give them courage, answers, hope and freedom from a lot of anxiety that I went through to get to the point of no return with my vision. If this book can reach and help even just one or a few people with eye issues to know that the end results of good vision, safer and healthier life are well worth the 10 minutes of surgery on each eye.

Day 10 I was rather nervous this day about the upcoming cataract surgery and lens implantation. My left eye vision was great, and I started to think that I could just live with my one bad eye and my one good eye. I was contemplating waiting longer and just retaining my vision the way it was. After all it was already so clear in my left eye how could I ask for more. I was afraid that going on to do the second eye would perhaps tempt fate and something bad would happen. But I realized that was sort of superstitious thinking. In the future I would have to have the second eye done anyhow. I was still getting multiple vision in my right eye. Occasionally my right eye would dominate while driving and I would get a flash of a multiple image. This disturbed me and I thought it was also dangerous. At this point I was glad surgery was imminent. I went for a 22-mile bike ride with my husband on Merritt Island. I this this was a great stress reliever and I was glad to know that I could still do long distance after forced medical rest.

Day 11 Monday 3/5 Bought new eye drops and prepped my right eye for second surgery. Tried to be calm and stay the course. Called my friends and talked to them about going through with the surgery. Listened to words of encouragement from them. Reviewed the process of the first surgery in my head so that I could keep myself calm and moving in that direction. This day was about holding my own and going forth into new direction of hope and success, with new light and a new vision for my life. I went for an 8-mile bike ride around Tropical Trail and my home as I knew that I would be on another week of rest following Tuesday's surgery.

Day 12 3/6/2019 Right Eye Tuesday Day of Second Surgery

Scheduled for 7:15am. I put drops in my left eye as usual and my husband drove me to the Surgical Center. After surgery on my right eye, I immediately noticed it was not as clear as the left eye. I was concerned that the wrong diopter strength lens was inserted. I was surprised how different the right and left eye are. At night I went outside, and I was seeing giant Ferris wheel like halos and concentric circles around lights and stars. I was worried and enchanted. I had never seen such incredibly beautiful spiderweb like images from lights even with multiple vision. On this day of surgery, I recorded an hourly detail of vision development although I was still dilated. I was sleeping once I got home, but when I woke up, I recorded what I saw.

9:00 am Very blurry

11:00 am whitish film over images, non-doubled or multiples

1:05 pm Hazy in right eye

2:00 pm Whitish haziness

3:00 pm Still hazy objects

4:00pm Hazy object albeit a bit clearer

5:00pm Vision still blurry in right eye

6:00pm Getting desperate that my right eye vision is not going to be as successful as the left eye.

7:00pm I went outside to see the streetlights. I almost freaked out until I made myself laugh it off. I was seeing enormous giant Ferris wheels around every streetlamp on my drive. This was way "better" than anything that I had with my normal lenses. I was about to cry and throw in the towel. In September of 2018, I swam the 9-mile swim to the Alligator Lighthouse of Islamorada and back to shore. I was dodging moon jellies but still managed to get stung about 20 times. I know exactly what these large circular razor-edged moon jellies can do and look like under water. I was seeing moon jellies in the sky now too. I got through the pain of multiple, multiple stings and did not give up till I swam back to shore after circum-swimming the lighthouse. By the time I got back, only two of those jellyfish stings stayed with me. I found my aloe and soothed my wounds. I just heard my dad's voice in my head, "you must be patient, the vision will come in. It takes time. It can take four weeks till it settles in properly." When he first told me that I almost cried in disbelief. My left eye was perfect, nearly so, the second day. And from the first day, I could see images sharply even though the white film covered. But the ophthalmologist had said that it was highly unusual that the vision is perfect so fast. So, I thought okay, I'll wait another week. I can see well already. Its just going to get better. Think positive!!

Day 13 Wednesday One day post-operative appointment. My vision in the right eye was still not as clear as the left eye. There were floaters in my left eye but not in the right eye. Did not get good rest as my son was stung by 10 wasps and had to go to the ER. Computer vision good. Driving fine except that eyes were dry which was creating halos around lights at night. I put in preservative free lubricating eye drops which helped a lot to reduce the halos. We drove to ER and then to CVS. I was able to read at a distance the prescription, but not very clearly with both eyes. So, I used my left eye. The giant Ferris wheel like concentric circles around lights were gone.

Day 14 Thursday 3/7 Supposed to be a rest day but son had to stay home from school. I was highly preoccupied with his medical health and emotional wellbeing. I monitored his welts from the wasp stings, equivocated about giving him pain killers, bought cold packs for him to put on his stings, kept him resting, cleaned house, washed clothes; all but rest! My eyes were functioning fine though. My vision was clear during the day inside.

Day 15 Friday Supposed to be a rest day but son had to stay home from school once again. We went to Walmart and my vision was getting pretty good. I was happy. I could read all the signs above the aisles. My brain and my vision were reconnecting in that I was able to process a lot more details. I could perceive my environment so much more again. The speed at which I was able to process jumped rapidly. I felt like I was about 20 years old again in terms of seeing and analyzing my environment. It felt awesome.

Day 16 Saturday 3/9/2019. I participate in a Community Band of Brevard County and play the flute. I went to dress rehearsal at 9:30 am till 12 noon. I was able to play and read the music from the normal distance on the music stand. Previously, I had to sit very close to the stand and peer at the sheet music. It's a good thing I'm not a trumpet player, as I never would have been able to see the page, sitting far away. As I was nearly blind, notes were blurry, some notes would white out as I was reading them; so, I might miss that note altogether. But now with new multi-focal lenses I can see, look ahead, process the meaning of the note, process the articulation of the note, count much better, and process the music much faster. I think this will do wonders for my music development and flute playing in the community band. At the dress rehearsal, the fluorescent lights in the room did bother my head and vision. My vision was shaky and glary.

At certain times I put my hands on the sides of my temples. This calmed and steadied my vision. Our concert was the next day in the afternoon at the Merritt Island High School auditorium. I had to decide whether to play. I had continued to practice my music throughout this process, only missing a few rehearsals. I felt 90% comfortable with the music and performing. However, from previous concerts, I knew the stage lights in the auditorium were particularly penetrating. I had two piccolo pieces to play, so I didn't want to let the band down.

After rehearsal we went to Walmart and my friend Don showed me some sunglasses which also had +2.0 readers. I can now use these glasses to go kayaking and read my Garmin Fenix and my Garmin GPSMAPS 78SC. Some of the fonts on my Fenix are small and right now still challenging to perceive. With these sunglasses, Don solved my problem. That night I did have a radiating pain throughout the right side of my head. It just passed through and did not stay or recur. It felt like a web of pain and then it dissolved.

Day 17 Sunday March 10, 2019 Concert Day! I invited my friend Don and my son to the concert. I drove there, errantly going to the rehearsal hall first. Realizing my mistake when the gates were locked, I did however see a new Lutheran church, Faith Lutheran which I decided was calling our name. We then drove to the high school. I went in, curious to see how my new vision would be able to handle the stage lights. I was glad since I was able to see everyone and the conductor. Just from on stage, oh boy those lights were super bright. The previous concert I must have been blind or clouded up to not notice how intolerably bright they were. I needed to adjust my music stand and gaze slightly downward to not have the bright lights glaring my vision.

I sit in the first row. So, we get the brightest of the lights directed at us. I sit next to a clarinet player. He is always taking note of things. I had told him of my lens implants. Today he decided to mention to me that the size of my eyes was slightly different. He observed that my right eye was open more than my left eye. Later when I looked in the mirror, I could see what he meant. My right eye was not closing as much, and my left eye was contracting around the eye socket. He said he only noticed since he always sits in that seat next to me. He said it wasn't totally obvious. However, I now recall that the scrub nurse in the OR really cleaned my eye cavity prior to surgery. My eye was already numbed so I didn't feel any pain, but I could tell that she was scraping or rubbing my eye socket. She kept apologizing to me as she was doing it. I wondered why she kept doing it if she had to apologize for her actions. So, I am thinking that she may have overstretched my right eye lid during pre-ops to surgery.

Well I was able to play in the concert. I played my piccolo parts in Choclo, Danzas Caribe and Stars and Stripes Forever. I played my new gold flute for all the other pieces. During the concert my eyes were getting dry. I drank water but my vision was still starting to shake a bit. At intermission, I put lubricating drops in each eye. This helped to settle my vision and I was able to play the second half of the concert. I assume this shaking is part of the adjusting and lens adaptation process following surgery. After all there is a silicone lens implanted into each eye.

I keep having to remind myself of this as so far, I have very little pain or discomfort associated with these surgeries. My vision is developing day by day. Sometimes I have a mild point of pain or pressure feeling in my left eyeball. But I had this already prior to the surgery and it comes and goes. The doctor said that dry eyes causes this and to put lubricating drops in. I also have a floater which moves around my left eye sometimes causing distortion in my vision. One of my doctors said not to worry about the floaters they will go away.

Driving home again from the restaurant, I noticed that my absolute best vision is in the far distance. I can see freighters with greater detail out in the ocean. Across the river I can see the condominium buildings, each tiny house on the waterfront, and the moon as a single moon in crescent phase? At the restaurant I could see people's eyes, what people look like again, read the menu, see the food, read the bill. But I looked up at the moon, half cringing that I would see multiple images of the crescent. I turned and looked away. There was a slight doubling of the crescent. I could not look anymore. It was so painful to see this and to think that I was never going to have proper sharp clear vision again. I just went home and went to sleep, depressed.

Day 18 On Monday morning, I awoke thinking perhaps the concert, the drinks, going out to Grills Riverside after, the fun perhaps was too much since surgery had only been six days prior. So, I opened my eyes and found that after adjusting to daylight, each eye was still doing well. Thank goodness God! Today, my left eye, the one that had the first lens implanted was focusing the near vision better. It has been 13 days since the first surgery and my eyes are working well together. The best vision I am having is with both eyes. My vision at the desktop computer is very clear. However, light is still causing reverberations in my brain and sometimes I get flashes. But if I close my eyes or hold my head in my hands, I can still these effects. I just discovered that if I sit back a little bit farther from the computer screen, this reverberation stops. I am adjusting the distances of my tech devices now too. I now hold my cell phone at arm's length in reading text or emails. Tonight, I was outside, and I looked up at the sky and there was a single sliver of a crescent moon. I was elated! The vision that I had of the moon was nearly telescopic. It looked as if I was looking through a telescope! It was beautiful and clear! I took another look and saw the shadow of the dark part of the moon along with the crescent. Wow, this was worth waiting another day for! I can't wait till full moon! This month I will see one circular moon. I haven't seen that in two years!

Day 19 My son came home from school and wanted to go to Best Buy to get a drone. I relented because he is great at flying drones. On the way home, I noticed that my night vision was clear, and I had minimal halos on cars I was following. I still saw some halos on oncoming traffic. Later when we arrived home, got out of the car and I glanced at the moon. It was a perfect crescent. It was so beautiful and crystal clear! I was elated and in awe of how good my vision was getting. I had forgotten to put my eye drops in three times by 11pm, so I did a double dose within ten minutes to make sure that I could fill in my chart properly.

Day 20 March 13, 2019 One-week post-operative check up on right eye. I put in my eye drops this morning late, since I had a headache and I had put in two doses late last night. At the check-up I discussed a shimmering of light that I see with the doctor. He mentioned that the IOL is in a capsule and can move around until it settles in the space. I think this may be what is causing the movement of light that I perceive. Even though my right eye was dilated during the check up, I was still able to drive myself home wearing my sunglasses. I kept the sunglasses on well into the evening though as I noticed that my eyes were still rather sensitive to the light up until sunset around 7:30pm. I was on my phone and playing a game on an app. I noticed that my up-close vision was blurrier than it had been before. I think the glaucoma drops and the dilating drops reduced my vision again. Around 11pm I went outside again to view the moon. I was so happy again to see how clear the second quarter moon is looking. The stars were also clear and not doubled. They had ever so tiny halos around them but those were less than before. I was very encouraged when the doctor and his technicians mentioned that vision continues to improve 12 weeks from surgery and even further on. At this point, I can return to the swimming pool and to kayaking. I can wear goggles again, whereas early on after the surgery, the pressure on my head would have been too much. Frankly, I have been out of the pool so long now, I hope I remember how to swim! I need to start training for my June 1, 2019 12-mile swim around Key West!

Day 21 In one week, I will be able to discontinue the eye drops in my left eye. I am very excited about this as it is rather difficult to maintain all these eye drops. From the anti-inflammatory steroidal drops, I get a postnasal drip which is unpleasant. Also, the burning of these eye drops does not always subside even with using the preservative free eye lubricant drops. It bothers me that I need to continue with all these eye drops, but I will continue to apply the proper dosages. Both my parents continue to encourage me to see the drops to the end of the prescribed duration to have the best results. I certainly do not want to jeopardize my vision for the rest of my life for the sake of convenience. I thought about going swimming or kayaking today but took the dogs to the beach instead. It was warm and windy, but my eyes were fine, and I did not get any sand in them, although I sat down on the beach and my dog Lucky decided to kick sand up at that very moment! I think my return to normal life is imminent! This time it is way cooler though. I don't have to wear glasses, except sunglasses anymore! Awesome! I may try going kayaking tomorrow. I am a little wary about the water from the Indian River Lagoon or the Banana River. The doctor said the incisions have closed, but I may still wait a little longer as I was reading on a UK website that swimming is not recommended for 4-6 weeks after surgery is complete. So, I had surgery on February 21, 2019 and March 5, 2019. Four weeks would be April 5 and six weeks will be April 19, 2019. Today is March 14, 2019. I wonder why the doctor said it was alright to return to swimming. He mentioned that I have the same level of risk of infection now that I had prior to surgery. I have either healed up very quickly or the phacoemulsification performed is slightly different in the USA than in the UK. In my eyes they made two tiny incisions without using stitches. I am now considering getting a VASA swim trainer to resume my swim training sooner. While I love the time off, I won't be ready for the

June 1 swim around Key West if I sit out too long now! I realize that the containers of ice cream I am eating outweigh the barbells I am lifting!

Day 22 Today I awoke, sat up in bed and strangely enough saw stars, lights floating around my vision. There were twinkling lights just in front of me. Immediately I was concerned! But I blinked a couple of times and they were gone! So, I went to put in the eye drops. Any thought of early discontinuation of the drops just vanished. Then after I input the drops, my vision was a bit whitish. I went outside and it was very sunny. I wore sunglasses, but I removed my sunglasses once in a store and still thought things looked a bit whitish.

Day 23 When I wake up in the morning, it takes a few seconds for my vision to clear. I think I have a floater in my left eye which sometimes creates a shadowiness. But if I blink a couple of times then it is gone. Today my vision was bit whitish again but less so and only in my left eye.

Day 24 Again when I awoke, it took a few seconds for my eyes to achieve the perfect clarity that I like to see. I use the bedside Bose clock radio digital display for my morning vision test. If I glance at those red numbers and they are clear, then all is well. If not, I close the right eye and then peer through the left to determine the sharpness of the left eye vision. Then I do the same clearness vision test with my right eye. When I do this, my eyes then start working more. I get much clearer vision when I then use both eyes again to sight. I am extremely picky with my vision. I venture to say that any ordinary person would find the initial waking up clarity to be satisfactory.

Day 25 Today as I awoke, I did my digital clock vision test again. It was about the same as yesterday. The right eye today was clearer than the left eye. I realize there is a role that other parts of my eye play in the focusing of an image, besides my lens. As I wake up more parts, such as the retina, begin to function more. I continue to use the drops three times a day. I still have enough drops in the bottles, but I am running low on the left eye pink top bottle of Ketorolac. If I completely run out, I will use the other pink top bottle first before I get another refill. Here is another picture of my eye drop station which I set up in my bathroom.

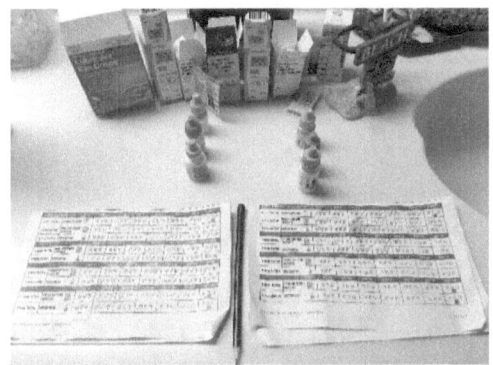

Figure 4 Using three drops 1 day prior to and 1 week after surgery

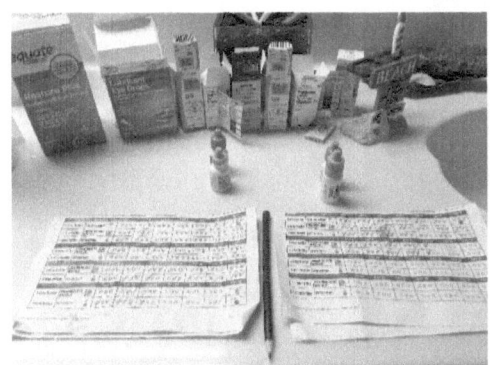

Figure 5 Using two drops two to four weeks after surgery

After the 28-day required eye drop schedule, the doctor said that I could still get an infection. Just before I run out, I will get one more refill of the eye drops just to have on hand in case an infection should arise. I went to look at the pool and looked at the kayak put in at the pool pavilion. Soon I will be going swimming again. Tomorrow I will look for my goggles. It will be momentous. I went for a beach walk and two bike rides.

Day 26 Left eye – 3 days of drops remaining and right eye 15 days of drops remaining. Today I am still noticing a whitishness in my right eye. Every now and then during the day my vision gets slightly blurred. If I blink a few times, I can get it to clear up again. My left eye is still more yellowish and has a floater in it. The lens in my right eye looks newer than the one in my left eye.

The blurriness goes in and out. Overall my vision is still very good with both eyes seeing together. I try to read every minute print and although I am capable of this, I think it tires out my eye musculature. So perhaps I am just eye tired. Today I was writing music, playing the piano, reading minute print on packaging, made pizza, framed and hung art on our house walls. I feel alive again and very happy to be functioning so well. I went to look at the pool, found my swim caps, looked at the kayak put in at the pool pavilion. Soon I will be going swimming again. Tomorrow I will look for my goggles. It will be momentous. I went for a beach walk and two bike rides. I found my swim caps and bathing suits. I am so excited to be getting back to my swim training and kayaking soon. I have had almost a month-long break now! Today was windy and cool, now great for either swim or kayak.

Day 27 On my first day back kayaking I will kayak 2020. If its good weather I will swim 2,020 meters (40-60 minutes) and then kayak 20.20 miles (5-6 hours on the water). Today Is a rainy day again. I probably will go for a walk in between rain showers. Upon awaking, my reading vision again took time to focus in clearly. The font size on my phone is tiny though. Most people would need a magnifying glass to read it. My mid distance and far vision are fine. The clarity is enhanced today, and I don't see the whitishness now. I feel like being very productive. I will hang more art on my home walls. I really feel good with my new lenses. There is a wonderful newness to my spirit. Could new eyesight really bring spiritual renewal too? Wow another great benefit of having 20/20 vision again.

I dutifully am using the eye drops still. But both the Ketorolac and the Prednisone are anti-inflammatory steroids. I am getting discomforting postnasal drip again which feels like it is numbing my anterior nasal chamber as the drip is going onto the back of my tongue and has a very unpleasant taste. It is mixing with my saliva and coming forward in my mouth too. My two front teeth and my nose feel numb also. I wish I could just stop taking these. I have not had any infection or inflammation as far as I can tell. There has been no severe pain, no redness no lasting pain and very little discomfort over the past two to three weeks in this healing process. I have experienced this postnasal drip when I have had to apply eye drops to both eyes simultaneously. I sometimes apply the drop sequentially, one after another. When I do the left eye first and wait, then do the right eye, it is better. I think I will go back to doing that. There is just too much liquid going into the eyes. Also, I used the Equate preservative free drop to stem the stinging from the Prednisone, which added even more liquid to the eye. This may have increased the flowing through my nasal chambers and into my throat. I thought the Equate would give me a headache, but it did not.

Day 28 (March 20,2019) This morning I awoke early but did not want to start the drops at 5:35 am. I waited till about 7:30 am and then put drops in my eyes simultaneously again. This time I got a pretty good burn from the prednisolone ophthalmic solution, so broke out another preservative lubricating drops very quickly. Adding the lubricating drops stops the burning or stinging sensation as the solution floods my eyes, mixing with the prednisolone. It is now 9 am and I am seeing very well. My vision is mostly stable and clear. Sitting at the computer I get a little shakiness but no whitishness today. I am feeling confident about my vision and getting back into doing things. Yesterday and today I am framing my artwork and hanging art on our walls. We moved into our new house June 2018, so it's about time to get it decorated with the art we have.

Day 29 March 21, 2019 I am so excited again about seeing things in life! Tonight, is the Supermoon, the Worm Moon. I could see the moon perfectly clearly, in a clear sky. It's so fantastic! I can see mare and craters on the moon. I took my telescope out on the front lawn and sighted the moon. I even had a mini star party with my husband my son Rex! We all took turns looking at the moon craters trough the scope. My son brought the Nikon and the tripod. He took pictures straight on. Later I had the idea to take picture of the night sky supermoon with the clouds encircling. There was a purplish and rainbow effect of the clouds surrounding the moon. I am very happy and excited to be able to utilize my telescope and my 40x telephoto camera again, view beautiful sights and try to take the pictures that I see! I think I was successful in capturing the moments I felt were amazing and beautiful. There truly can be beauty, wonder, amazement in every moment of life. We just need to be on the lookout for it. And waiting with a camera, a pencil and sketch pad or canvas and brush to note it down! Thank you so very much to God and all the doctors and nurses, friends, family, acquaintances and people that I met who have been impactful in my decision to have lens replacements. My world has truly opened again. Where I once thought despair was the road to take, I now know differently. There are solutions to grave problems in life. We must keep searching till we find them. Now every day I can go out and see the moments of life again as they unfold before me!

Day 30 March 22, 2019 Today has been my worst day yet. I woke up with a headache and pain centered in my forehead area. The pain lasted all day. I took some Tylenol late to see if that would help. I had to take three 500mg before I felt relief. This is unusual for me. One pill usually does the trick. On the bright side, we did go to Cocoa Beach for a beach day! We had a good time swimming in the ocean. I did not submerge yet and wore my mirrored Vanquisher Speedo goggles. I just played in the waves and my son used his surfboard, surfing the waves. We all went for a beach walk about 1.5 miles roundtrip. I was happy to be by the ocean again. I swam a short pace of breaststroke. We then all went to Steak and Shake expecting to get great burgers. I mistakenly ordered Buffalo Ranch Burger. Yuk! I also ordered the All-American burger. That was good! Yum! So, we drove home, and I still had a headache and my eyes were quite dry. I put in lubrication drops which helped. This headache lasted all day.

I drove my dogs to small beach at the end of our road for a walk. Then we drove over to Canova Beach dog park. It was still dusk, so we went on and walked up and down just the small section for dogs. My headache had lessened a bit. My cute dogs stuck their heads out the window when I rolled them down. They love going for rides. It was dark on the way back. My night vision is still somewhat a bother since I saw the spider web giant halos on red, yellow and some white lights. Car headlight are made of all sorts of different types of lights as some produce halos and others looks plain and normal. At one moment I even thought I saw a double vision of a headlight! Oh boy I was getting upset now! But I blinked and it went away and never came back.

Later however, I tried to sleep but was in such pain it was unbearable. The vision in my left eye seemed to be lessened and somewhat blurred. I took a Claritin since I was sneezing and felt some sinus pressure. I also added two more Tylenol. I finally fell asleep around 11pm.

Day 31 March 23, 2019 OMG!!! I did not wake up till 1:30 pm! My son came in and said he wanted to go to the beach again surfing. I do not have a headache today! I feel a slight pain in my left eye that shoots through my eye occasionally, around 1:55 pm. But that went away to as it was momentary.

My vision is very nice today clear and clean. So far, I just have a bit of sinus discomfort with slight pressure.

Chapter 10

The Reward of Restored Eyesight and Return to Productive Life

I am so thankful that my beautiful vision is restored through so much help from so many people. My vision is wonderfully clean in comparison to what it was prior to surgery. There are no multiples of any objects or lights anymore, colors appear very normal, sunsets have one setting sun and an atmospheric haze but nothing highly dramatic as from when my cataracts where splitting light all over the place. There are some small halos around lights still, but I hope these will minimize and go away over time. My world is very calm again. The sunsets are very pretty. A few days ago, there was a brushstroke of purple and pink in the sky at dusk. It was about the cleanest brushstroke I had seen in about two years. I am very thankful for my renewed 20/20 vision. I had practically resigned myself, prior to surgery, to adapting to a life of near blindness, expecting my vision to go from bad to worse. Daily I needed to think of new ways to compensate for the distortions in my vision I was experiencing. Fortunately for me, my parents and the many other people that have been helped my phacoemulsification and IOL implantation, we now have perfect 20/20 eyesight or nearly so. We no longer need to spend a lot of time making up mental compensations and mental translations for a distorted environmental input.

There is a tremendous amount of stress relief that goes along with having 20/20 vision again. I feel so much calmer and more peaceful. In shedding all this visual based stress, I have a great sense of relief and feeling of well-being now. Before I used to run into things around the house, such as walls, corners and trip over shower stalls. I would have to get very close to objects to see what they were. Now every day I can open my eyes to a clear world. I can see far in the distance but also in the intermediate distance. Everything is clear. My near vision is clear at arm's length. If I hold things any closer though it is blurry at a font size of 12 or smaller. If I increase the font size, then I can see it clearly. In eating, if I sit too close to my food, it is not totally clear! I need to push the plate away slightly, then it is clear. But I perceive this as a definite benefit to my weighty situation. Being calmer and pushing my plate away from me can only have slimming benefits. Another improvement via my new 20/20 vision.

There is a definite adjustment period to my new 20/20 eyesight. Now I am readjusting my physical behaviors since I can see high amount of detail in distances. I can view from afar many new things. The horizon in my area is an interesting one. I do not have to be right near things anymore to see what they are.

I can see that this 20/20 eyesight can come in handy in playing my favorite sports again. Open water swimming in the beautiful blue ocean, sea kayaking across new channels, skiing, playing golf and tennis again, bird watching, even travelling to see new biomes or working on a new career are some of the many things that I can enjoy again! I am so excited about my eyesight; I am even considering a new career as an airline pilot since I now have 20/20 vision. I am also thinking of setting up my telescope at nights again. The sky is just beckoning. I feel that I need to give back something for this second chance at life!

I also have a renewed confidence level as a mom. Now I can say to my son, "don't worry, I got this! I have 20/20 vision again!" The other day he asked me if my vision really was much better. I told him I can certainly see everything extremely well. I think it put a renewed level of confidence in him too. Having a mom who could not see well, fell on a ski slope due to misreading the ice, stopped driving at night, bumped into things around the house, could not see my son at his Winter concert, had to ask my husband which one was my son on the lacrosse field and the baseball field (ugh), had to ask to be led to places in a store because she could not see the store signage all put a damper on his life for the last two years. But no more! Now if I trip and fall, it's because I am not looking where I am going, not because I can't see it! I do not need help shopping anymore. I can read the signs all the way to the back of the store. I can't wait to see my son in his next concert! I am excited about playing golf and tennis again! No more blurs in the distance or double and triple balls coming at me or in the air on the serve! I am back thanks to the many people involved in my vision restoration!

    I also have a renewed confidence level in myself as a traveler, swimmer and kayaker. I am glad that I stopped travelling for a while. I put on hold going to events, going skiing, going to bucket list places like the Maldives, Madagascar, Tahiti, the Florida Everglades, the Bay of Fundy and Nova Scotia, Alaska, the Dolomites, Ushuaia, Patagonia, Bariloche, New Zealand, and Australia. So many places I realize that I still want to see! Now when I do resume going places, I will enjoy it because I will be able to safely and clearly view my surroundings.

During this whole process, we moved to Florida. This move happened as my eyesight was getting worse. Knowing that we were going to live on a nature preserve in a quiet area gave me a great sense of relief and safety. We were leaving the NJ/NY tristate area with its millions of people and cars, lights, headlights, headache producing, eyesight distorting and disturbing reality. A quiet more rural area was a haven for life with my diminishing eyesight. I was becoming quite depressed about moving to such a pretty area only to lose my eyesight! But now that my vision has been restored to a perfect 20/20, an entirely new benefit has come about. I can now truly see the beauty of the nature around me. And I can now explore my new world. There are so many nice places to see in Florida that I can start a bucket list with just my new home state first! It's a wonderful life! Thank you, God and all the doctors, nurses, physicians' assistants, ophthalmology and optometry techs, surgical counselors, administrators, brothers, friends, family, mom and dad, husband and son and our two doggies! I can see again! Thank God!

Terms

Phaco-emulsification

Intra-Ocular Lens (IOL)

Prism Glasses

Cataract Surgery

Cataract

References

1. Wikipedia-

https://en.wikipedia.org/wiki/Phacoemulsification

2. Eye Institute of Medicine and Surgery

http://www.seebetterbrevard.com/index

3. Charles Kelman, M.D.

http://www.laskerfoundation.org/awards/show/phacoemulsification-for-outpatient-cataract-surgery/

Books by Pia Lord

Harvest While the Orchard is Aplenty

Rhapsody

Hearts Can Sing

Mind Over Matter

The American Baby Collection

Cato the Caterpillar

The Night the Moon Went Out

The Day the Sun Went Out

Let's Take a Trip in Our Spaceship

The Adventures of M.M. Music Mouse

Books by Pia Lord (continued)

Catskills in the Rocky Mountains

El Teide Canary Island Volcano

La Masca Gorge

The Upper Limit

Time Travel

Just Pia!

Five Days in Tenerife -A Canary Island Love Story

Return to the Sea

Return to the Sea II

Sunflowers of Sans Souci Oma's Garden

Maddy and Jane Go to the Opera

The Sun Rises in China (One Act Opera in Five Scenes)

Books by Rex Lord

The Applesauce is Lost

Let's Take a Trip in Our Spaceship

About the Author

Pia Lord has earned a M.S. in Space Studies from American Public University, (with Honors), a B.A. in Economics from Barnard College, a B.M. in Music from William Patterson University (with Honors), a Diploma in Voice Performance from Mannes College of Music Extension Division, and A. A. in Fine Arts (Music Option) from Anne Arundel Community College .She enjoys writing mostly novellas and sci-fi stories. She likes to travel but enjoys playing music on her piano and flute. For exercise she loves surf skiing, sailing and swimming on the Indian River Lagoon in her hometown in Florida.

www.ingramcontent.com/pod-product-compliance
Lightning Source LLC
Chambersburg PA
CBHW021438210526
45463CB00002B/569